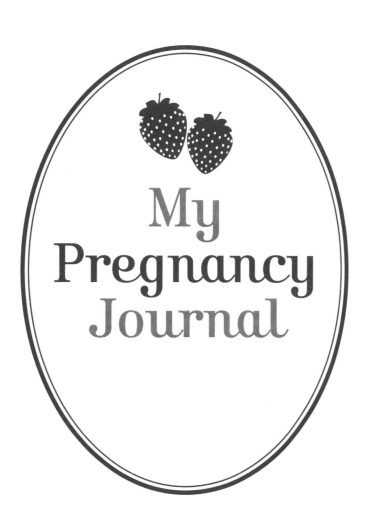

My
Pregnancy
Journal

THE EXPERIMENT

My Pregnancy Journal with Sophie la girafe

© 2014 SOPHIE LA GIRAFE All rights reserved
Modèle déposé / Design patent
Sophie la girafe© : Product protected by copyright
(by order of the Paris court of appeal dated 30 June 2000)

First published in France in 2014 as Mon Journal de
Grossesse Sophie la girafe® by Marabout.

Translation by Amy Butcher

The Experiment, LLC
220 East 23rd Street, Suite 600
New York, NY 10010-4658
theexperimentpublishing.com

This book contains the opinions and ideas of its author. It is intended to provide helpful and informative material on the subjects addressed in the book. It is sold with the understanding that the author and publisher are not engaged in rendering medical, health, or any other kind of personal professional services in the book. The author and publisher specifically disclaim all responsibility for any liability, loss, or risk—personal or otherwise—that is incurred as a consequence, directly or indirectly, of the use and application of any of the contents of this book.

The Experiment's books are available at special discounts when purchased in bulk for premiums and sales promotions as well as for fund-raising or educational use. For details, contact us at info@theexperimentpublishing.com.

ISBN 978-1-61519-234-2

Cover and text design by Marabout
Typeset by Christopher King

Manufactured in China
Distributed by Workman Publishing Company, Inc.
Distributed simultaneously in Canada by the University of Toronto Press

First printing: November 2014
10 9 8 7 6 5 4

My Pregnancy Journal

9 months of a woman's life . . .

9 months of changes to your
body, mind, and soul . . .

9 months of precious details
you'll never want to forget.

This pregnancy journal is the story of you
and your growing baby.

It's a record of all your thoughts, feelings, and secrets,
both big and small, and filled with things you need to
know on your journey to motherhood. You can personalize
it by adding your own photos and other mementos, and
use it to prepare for the arrival of your baby.

Both a guide and a keepsake, this journal will be your
companion through every step of your pregnancy, and
you'll treasure the priceless memories it holds forever.

This is your personal diary,
so make it your own however you please!

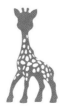

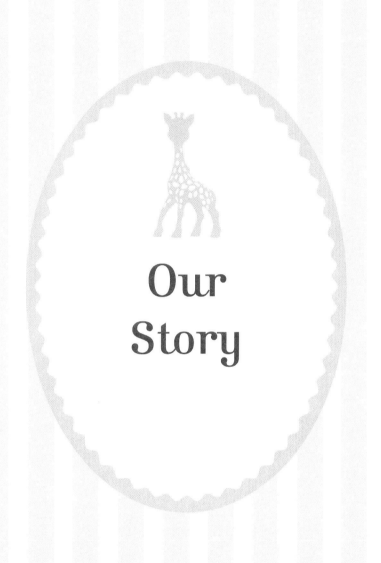

Our
Story

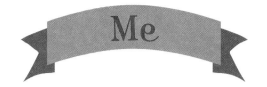

Me

My name is ....

I'm .... years old

I grew up in ....

I have .... brother(s)

I have .... sister(s)

My parents' names are

....

My siblings' names are

....

My mother's best qualities:

....

....

My father's best qualities:

....

....

My fondest childhood memory:

....

....

My favorite games and toys:

....

....

My childhood heroes:

....

....

My favorite vacation spot:

....

The family traditions I'd like to continue:

....

....

....

....

My Personality Profile

If I were a color,
I would be ....

If I were a season,
I would be ....

If I were an animal,
I would be ....

If I were a flower,
I would be ....

If I were a tree,
I would be ....

If I were a city,
I would be ....

If I were a food,
I would be ....

If I were a drink,
I would be ....

If I were a TV show,
I would be ....

If I were a movie,
I would be ....

If I were a book,
I would be ....

If I were a superhero,
I would be ....

If I were a celebrity,
I would be ....

If I were a person from history,
I would be ....

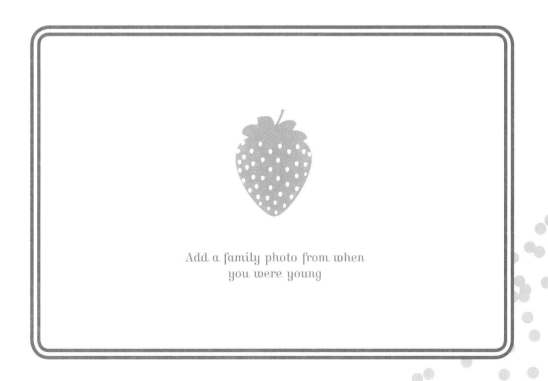

Add a family photo from when
you were young

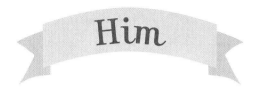

Him

His name is ....

He's .... years old

He grew up in ....

He has .... brother(s)

He has .... sister(s)

His parents' names are

....

His siblings' names are

....

His mother's best qualities:

....

....

His father's best qualities:

....

....

His fondest childhood memory:

....

....

His favorite games and toys:

....

....

His childhood heroes:

....

....

His favorite vacation spot:

....

The family traditions he'd like to
continue:

....

....

....

....

His Personality Profile

If he were a color,
he would be ....

If he were a season,
he would be ....

If he were an animal,
he would be ....

If he were a flower,
he would be ....

If he were a tree,
he would be ....

If he were a city,
he would be ....

If he were a food,
he would be ....

If he were a drink,
he would be ....

If he were a TV show,
he would be ....

If he were a movie,
he would be ....

If he were a book,
he would be ....

If he were a superhero,
he would be ....

If he were a celebrity,
he would be ....

If he were a person from history,
he would be ....

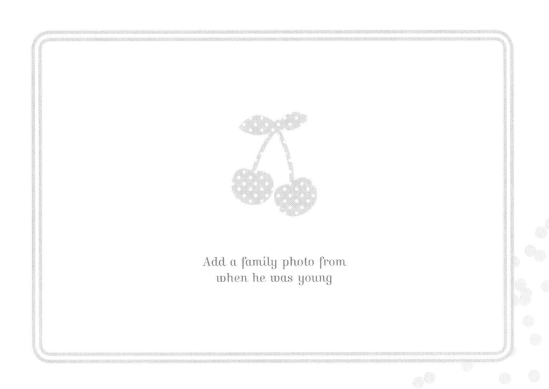

Add a family photo from
when he was young

How We Met

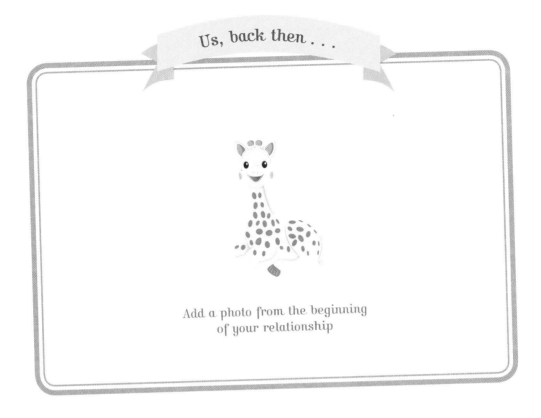

Us, back then . . .

Add a photo from the beginning
of your relationship

I was .... years old

He was .... years old

Our jobs at the time:

Me ....
....

Him ....
....

When did we meet?
....

Where did we meet?
....
....

How did it happen?
....
....
....
....
....

My first impression of him:
....
....
....
....
....

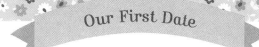
Our First Date

When did it happen?

....
....

Where did it happen?

....
....

How did it go?

....
....

What our parents said when they found
out we were together:

....
....
....
....
....

What our friends said when they found
out we were together:

....
....
....
....
....
....

Our Life Now

★ Just the Two of Us ★

What I do for a living: ....

What he does for a living: ....

We live in ....

In a ....

How a baby will change our lives:

....

....

....

★ Our Children ★

Our first child is named

....

and is .... years old.

Our second child is named

....

and is .... years old.

Our third child is named

....

and is .... years old.

Add a photo
of your children

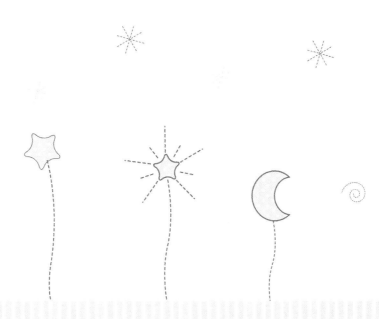

Add a photo of your
home sweet home

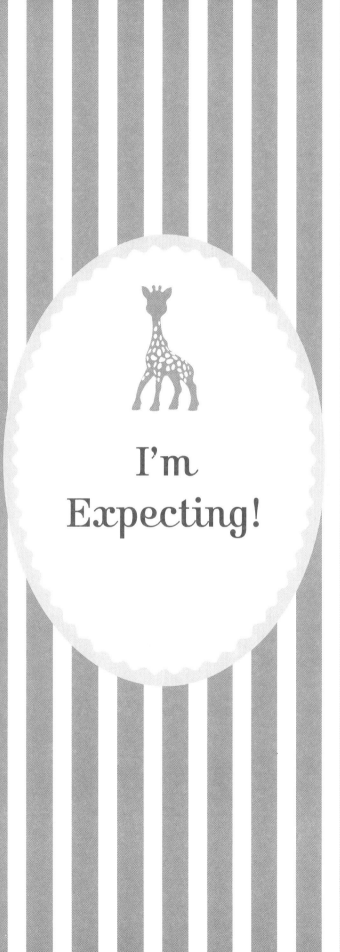

I'm
Expecting!

Dreams of Motherhood

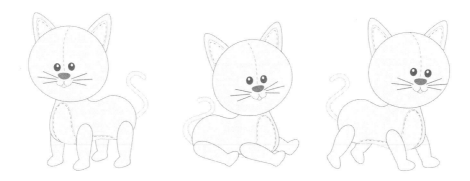

When I was young . . .

I wanted to have my first child at the age of .... years old.

I wanted .... children: .... boys and .... girls.

I wanted their names to be:

....

....

....

....

....

....

....

And Now . . .

When did I first begin thinking about having a baby?

....

....

Why?

....

....

....

How I envision myself as a mother: ....

....

....

....

....

....

....

....

....

....

....

....

....

....

The qualities I hope my baby will have:

....

....

....

....

....

....

What I hope my baby won't do:

....

....

....

....

....

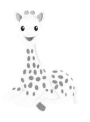

How It All
Started

I've been trying to have a baby since ....

How I prepared:

....
....
....
....

When do I think I conceived?

....

Where do I think I conceived?

....

I first had a feeling I was pregnant because:

....
....
....
....
....

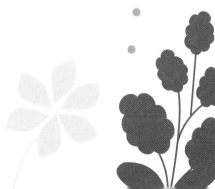

The Test!!!

When did I take the test?

....

Where did I take it?

....

Who waited for the result with me?

....

....

What I thought when I saw it was positive

O Do these things really work?

O Finally!!!

O No more mojitos

O No more sushi

O Am I going to get fat?

O ....

O ....

O ....

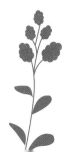

My First Reactions

Thoughts of Joy

- Finally!!!
- Whoa, this is actually happening!
- Imagine my mother's face when I tell her!
- ....
- ....
- ....
- ....
- ....

My Resolutions

- Save money!
- Lay off the junk food
- Stay active
- ....
- ....
- ....
- ....
- ....

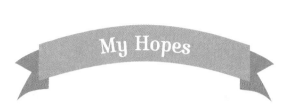

My Hopes

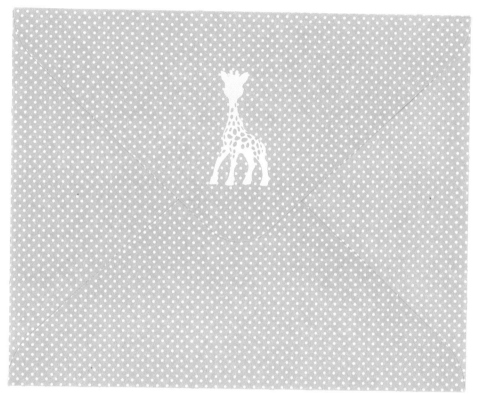

Dear Baby: Although you're not here yet, I want to tell you . . .

....

....

....

....

....

My Baby's Development

End of Month 1

...nnouncement on the
...ast page of the book!

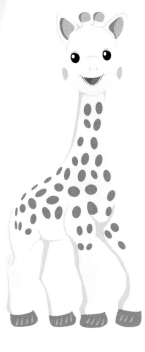

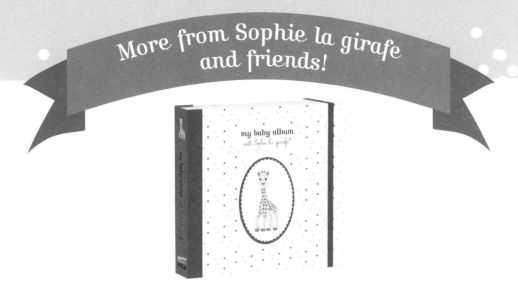
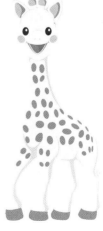

Add the

birth announcement

The first thing I did when I woke up:

O Touched my toes

O Took a shower

O Enjoyed some coffee

O Devoured an entire steak . . . rare, of course!

O ....

O ....

O ....

O ....

Today in national news . . .

....

....

....

....

....

....

....

Today in world news . . .

....

....

....

....

....

....

....

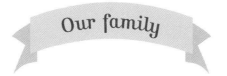

Our family

Add your first family photo

Here's how it all happened:

....
....
....
....
....
....
....
....
....
....
....
....
....
....

My baby!

Add a photo of
your baby

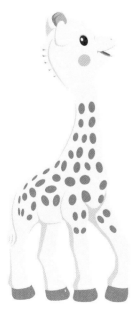

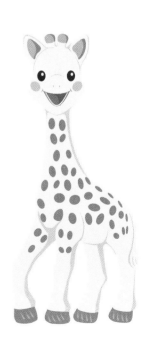

Name: ....

Place of birth: ....

Born on: ....

at .... a.m./p.m.

Length: .... in.

Weight: .... lbs.

How did I wait out my labor?

....
....
....
....
....
....
....
....

What was my labor like
until the delivery?

....
....
....
....
....
....

Add a photo from when
the excitement got started

What made me smile:

....
....
....
....
....

What stressed me out:

....
....
....
....
....

D-Day

Did I do anything special that day?

....
....
....
....

Some of the signs that I was in labor:

○ I had to go to the bathroom, a lot

○ My water broke

○ My stomach started cramping

○ Every little thing set me off

○ ....

○ ....

○ ....

What was Dad's reaction?

....
....
....
....

Welcome,
Baby!

The first time . . .

I couldn't wait to finally give birth

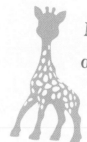

My belly became an obstacle

_____
_____
_____
_____
_____
_____
_____
_____

The last time . . .

I could put my shoes on
by myself

I could see my feet while
standing up

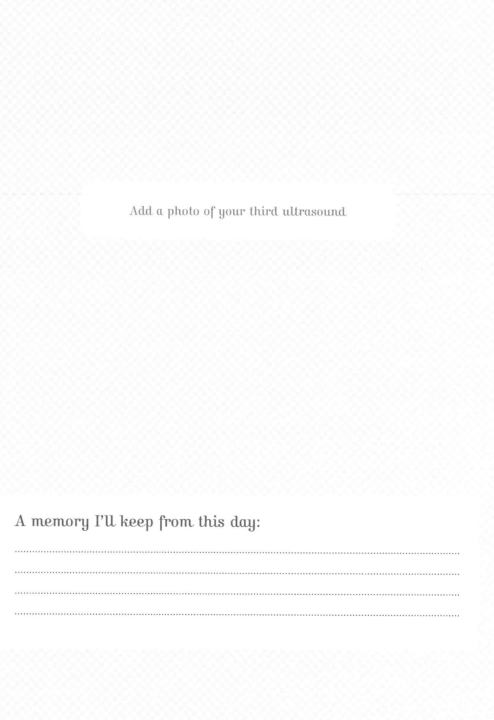

Add a photo of your third ultrasound

A memory I'll keep from this day:

....
....
....
....

The Doctor's Visit

When is it?

....

Where is it?

....

Who's coming with me?

....

What are my concerns?

....
....
....
....
....

What I learned:

....
....
....
....

My reaction:

....
....
....
....

Dad's reaction:

....
....
....
....

The Third Trimester

How will he participate in the delivery?

O By holding my hand

O By recording everything

O By coaching my breathing

O By whispering sweet nothings in my ear

O ....

O ....

O ....

O ....

Does he want to stay until the end?

....

Why?

....

....

Does he want to cut the cord?

....

Why?

....

....

How's Dad Doing?

How is he managing the stress?

○ By getting sympathy pains
○ By being overprotective
○ By throwing himself into his work
○ By renovating the entire house
○ ....
○ ....
○ ....
○ ....

His last-minute worries, both big and small:

○ What if she gives birth in the car?
○ What if I faint?
○ Will I get any sleep after the baby comes?
○ ....
○ ....
○ ....
○ ....

Is he ready to become a dad? Why?

....
....
....
....

What I didn't expect to happen:

The nice surprises:

....
....
....
....
....
....
....
....

The not-so-nice surprises:

....
....
....
....
....
....
....
....

Almost a dad!

Add the last photo of him
before he became a dad

People we need to tell . . .

Who will share the news?

My Birth Plan

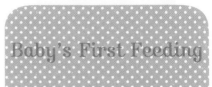

Baby's First Feeding

Breast or bottle?

....

Why?

....

....

For bottle feeding: Who
will give the bottle?

....

Why?

....

....

....

How I want to give birth:

- ○ With an epidural
- ○ Without an epidural
- ○ In water
- ○ With Dad by my side
- ○ ....
- ○ ....
- ○ ....
- ○ ....

My last-minute worries, both big and small:

- ○ What if I don't realize I'm in labor?
- ○ What if my doctor is out sick?
- ○ Will I need an episiotomy?
- ○ Will I have a Cesarean?
- ○ Will my stomach return to normal?
- ○ ....
- ○ ....
- ○ ....
- ○ ....

Things I need to bring for the hospital stay:

- My baby's outfit
- Comfortable clothes
- A sweater
- Socks and slippers
- My phone and phone charger
- Lotion
- A water bottle
- Loose change for vending machines
- ....
- ....
- ....
- ....

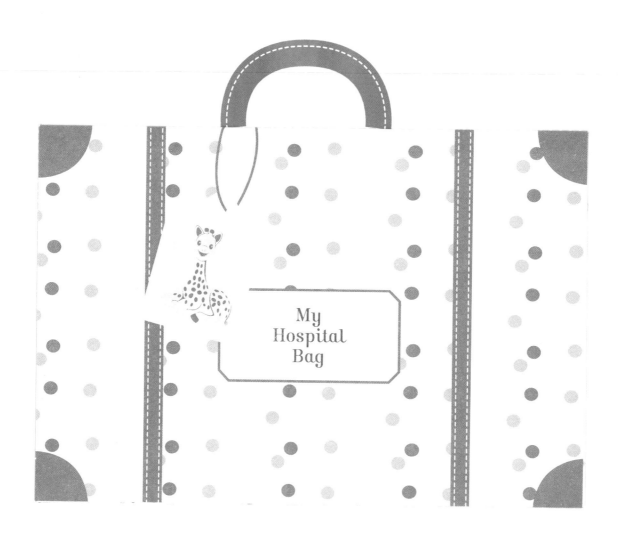

My Hospital Bag

My Hospital Bag

Baby's first outfit:

O 1 onesie

O 1 sleeper

O 1 warm sweater

O 1 soft cotton hat

O 1 pair of infant socks

O 1 newborn diaper

O ....

O ....

O ....

O ....

Add a photo of the outfit
you picked out for your baby

Why did I choose
these specific clothes?

O They belonged to my firstborn

O They're just too cute

O They're practical

O ....

O ....

O ....

O ....

The clothes I picked out for myself:

....

Why this outfit?..

....

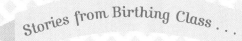

Stories from Birthing Class . . .

Tender or funny moments that occurred:

....
....
....
....
....
....
....
....
....
....

Class schedule:

....
....
....
....
....
....
....

....
....
....
....

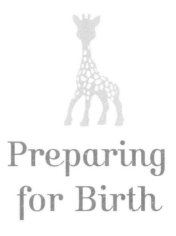

Preparing
for Birth

The birth classes I chose:

O Lamaze technique

O Alexander technique

O Bradley method

O HypnoBirthing

O None

O ....

O ....

O ....

Why did I choose this method?

....

....

....

How has it helped me prepare?

....

....

....

Who will be there during the delivery?

....

....

....

....

How will they help me?

....

....

....

....

....

Who do I think will come visit me afterward?

....

....

....

....

....

....

....

....

The Delivery Plan

Where will I give birth?

....

....

Why did I pick this place?

....

....

....

....

....

O Hospital birth?

O Home birth?

What do I think it will be like?

....

....

....

....

....

The Home
Stretch

Who will look after my baby when I go back to work?

....

How did I find this daycare service?

....

....

Why did I pick this daycare service?

....

....

What do I find reassuring about this daycare service?

....

....

Does anything worry me about this daycare service?

....

....

....

....

My plan so that no one at work forgets about me:

....

....

....

....

Balancing Family and Work

I start maternity leave on ..../........./.........

I'll stop working on .... because ....
....
....
....

Who will look after my other children during the delivery?
....

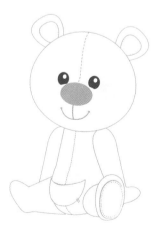

Who will help me after the delivery?

O The baby's dad

O My mother

O My cousin

O My retired neighbor

O ....

O ....

O ....

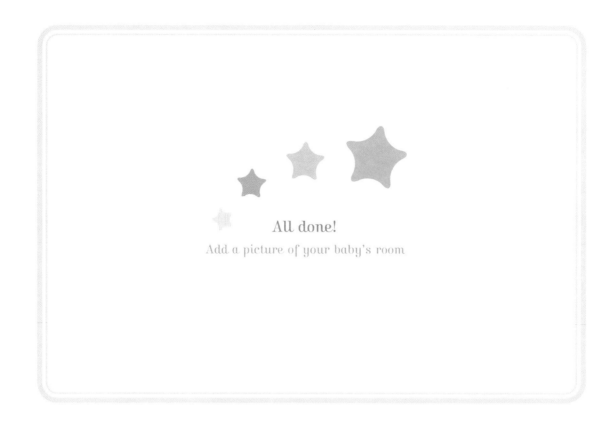

All done!

Add a picture of your baby's room

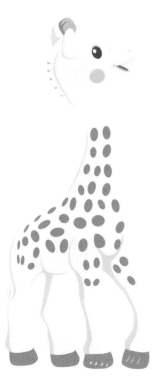

My little—and big—impulse buys!

○ An all-in-one convertible crib

○ A giant stuffed animal

○ A fancy baby carriage

○ An antique rocking chair

○ ....

○ ....

○ ....

○ ....

○ ....

○ ....

My Baby's Room

Who's going to paint it?

....
....
....

The toys waiting patiently
to be played with:

....
....
....
....
....
....
....

The color scheme I chose:

....

The theme I picked out:

....
....

Handcrafted from the heart!

Add a photo of something
that was created for
your baby's room

The furniture I picked out:

....
....
....
....
....
....
....
....
....

My Baby Registry

Where I'm registered:

....

What I asked for:

○ Car seat

○ Stroller

○ Crib and mattress

○ Bedding

○ Changing pad

○ Bath towels

○ Bottle warmer

○ Baby monitor

○ Baby carrier

○ Diaper bag

○ Mobile

○ ....

○ ....

○ ....

○ ....

○ ....

○ ....

○ ....

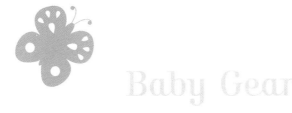

Baby Gear

What I thought the first time I set foot in a baby store:

....
....
....
....
....

Things I had to have:

....
....
....

Things that surprised me:

....
....
....

Things I wouldn't buy in a million years:

....
....
....
....

What I'm getting secondhand:

O A baby tub from ....

O A bottle sterilizer from ....

O A playpen from ....

O A highchair from ....

O ....

O ....

O ....

Clothes for baby's closet

The clothes that my baby will need

- O Onesies
- O Shirts
- O Pull-on pants or leggings
- O Sleepers
- O ....
- O ....
- O ....
- O ....
- O ....
- O ....
- O ....
- O ....
- O ....
- O ....
- O ....
- O ....
- O ....

- O Booties
- O Socks
- O Hats
- O Outerwear
- O ....
- O ....
- O ....
- O ....
- O ....
- O ....
- O ....
- O ....
- O ....
- O ....
- O ....
- O ....
- O ....

My Baby's Wardrobe

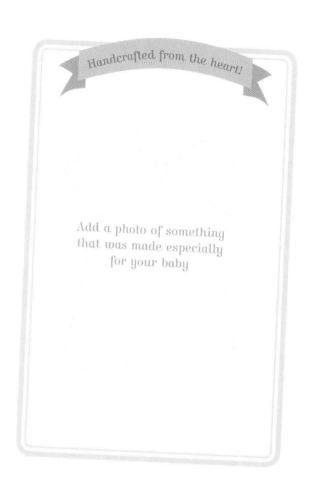

Handcrafted from the heart!

Add a photo of something
that was made especially
for your baby

Add a photo of your first
purchase for baby

The first baby clothes I bought:

....

I bought them at ....

When did I buy them? ....

My best finds:

....

....

....

....

Clothes people have given me that I absolutely love:

....

....

....

....

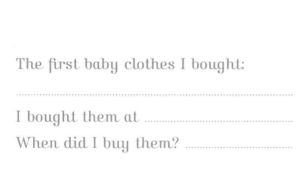

Add an invitation to your baby shower

Some memories from my baby shower:

....
....
....
....
....
....

My Baby Shower

Who hosted it?

....

When was it?

....

Where was it?

....

What was the theme?

....

Add a photo of the festivities

Add a photo of
the festivities

Who came?

....
....
....
....

What did we eat?

....
....
....

What games did we play?

....
....
....

The gifts I received:

....
....
....

Preparing
for Baby's
Arrival

The first time . . .

Someone on the bus offered me their seat

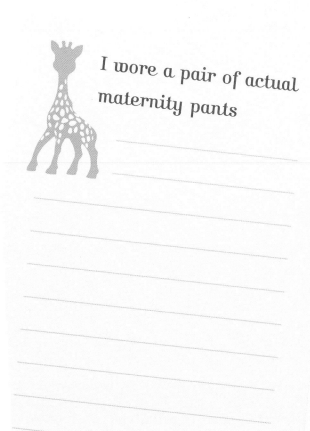

I wore a pair of actual maternity pants

_____

_____

_____

_____

_____

_____

_____

_____

_____

The last time . . .

I could go up the stairs
without needing to rest

I danced all night

_____

_____

_____

_____

_____

_____

_____

_____

_____

_____

Add a photo of your second ultrasound

A memory I'll keep from this day:

....

....

....

....

The Doctor's Visit

When is it?

....

Where is it?

....

Who's coming with me?

....

What are my concerns?

....

....

....

....

....

....

Will I ask about the baby's sex?

....

Is it a girl or a boy?

....

My reaction:

....

....

....

....

Dad's reaction:

....

....

....

....

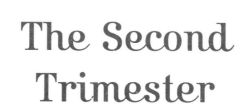

The Second
Trimester

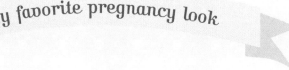
My favorite pregnancy look

Add a photo of you wearing
your favorite maternity outfit

Things that make me still feel fabulous:

○ Shirts that display my cleavage

○ Strappy sandals

○ Bright colors

○ Red lipstick

○ ....

○ ....

○ ....

○ ....

○ ....

○ ....

Things I can't live without:

○ My comfy maternity jeans

○ My stretchy T-shirts

○ My flip-flops

○ My cotton sweatpants

○ ....

○ ....

○ ....

○ ....

○ ....

○ ....

The first time I went shopping for maternity clothes:

....

....

What I bought:

....

....

My favorite brands:

....

....

....

Stores I don't dare to shop in anymore:

....

....

Maternity clothes that were passed down to me
that I wear a lot:

....

....

Maternity clothes that were passed down to me
that I rarely put on:

....

....

My Secrets for a Good Night's Sleep

○ I remove all screens, phones, and other distractions from my room.

○ I avoid caffeine, especially later in the day.

○ I don't take an afternoon nap and go to bed an hour earlier instead.

○ I do yoga, relaxation exercises, meditation, or tai chi.

○ I avoid drinking too many fluids in the evening.

○ I don't exercise in the evening.

○ For supper, I eat light.

○ I don't surf the internet in the evening.

○ I always go to bed at the same time.

○ I stick to the same bedtime routine every night.

○ I slowly and firmly massage my head for a full minute.

○ I put a sachet of dried lavender in my pillowcase.

○ I relax by putting a heating pad on my back every night.

○ I put up blackout curtains in my room.

○ I sleep with an eye mask.

○ I sleep with earplugs.

○ I try to sleep on my left side (to help with blood circulation).

○ I surround myself with pillows.

○ Instead of stressing out when I can't fall asleep, I read a bit.

○ ....

○ ....

My Sleeping Habits

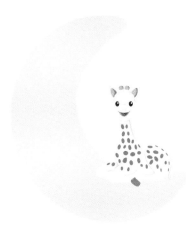

Before I needed .... hours of sleep every night

Now I need .... hours of sleep every night

To be well-rested,

I go to bed at .... p.m.

and wake up at .... a.m.

My favorite sleeping position:

....

....

My craziest dreams:

....

....

....

....

....

Nightmares that have me freaked out:

....

....

....

....

....

Nausea

o Drink a glass of water upon waking.

o Drink a glass of seltzer water.

o Drink lemon juice mixed with hot water and honey.

o Drink lemon juice mixed with cold seltzer water and a pinch of ground ginger.

o Eat often, but not a lot.

o On an empty stomach, nibble plain cookies, oat crackers, or rice cakes.

o Avoid dairy products.

o Choose neutral-tasting foods: white meat, pasta, rice, etc.

o Go outside to get some air or open the windows.

o Avoid wearing clothes that are too tight around the waist.

o With your thumb, firmly massage the center of your right wrist, just under your hand.

Gastric reflux

o Eat five to six small meals instead of three large ones.

o Eat meals sitting down, in a calm environment, and on a regular schedule.

o Eat slowly and chew each bite thoroughly.

o Avoid eating foods that are too hot or too cold.

o Avoid fats and dishes that are very rich.

o Avoid strong spices and peppers.

o Season dishes with mild flavors, like parsley, basil, vanilla, cinnamon, etc.

o Avoid acidic fruits (citrus).

o Never go to bed right after a meal.

o Exercise.

o Sleep slightly elevated (with pillows).

o Avoid leaning over (no housework!).

o Avoid carrying things that are too heavy (no groceries!).

o Dissolve a small amount of baking soda in water as an antacid (best not taken with meals).

o Take Maalox or Gaviscon (with your doctor's okay).

Itchy skin
(or to avoid stretch marks)

o Avoid gaining too much weight by exercising and eating healthfully.

o Stay hydrated by drinking water.

o Massage your belly, breasts, and buttocks every day with sweet almond oil.

o Variation 1: Give yourself a daily massage with organic olive oil.

o Variation 2: Give yourself a daily massage with Shea butter.

o Variation 3: Give yourself a daily massage with massage oil.

o Have your doctor prescribe a vitamin A skin treatment.

When do I feel my best?

O When I'm sleeping

O When I'm with friends

O When I'm exercising

O When I've had my daily dose of chocolate

O When ....

O When ....

O When ....

O When ....

O When ....

O When ....

O When ....

O When ....

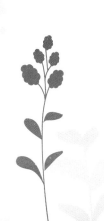

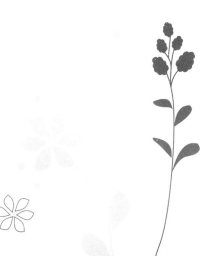

Smells I can't stand:

O Coffee   O Lemon-scented
O Body odor   dish soap
O Air freshener   O Seafood
O ....
O ....
O ....
O ....

My annoying symptoms:

O I'm itchy everywhere
O My stomach feels heavy
O I'm nauseated all the time
O My legs are swollen
O My face has broken out
O ....
O ....
O ....
O ....

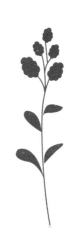

What's different compared to my previous pregnancies?
Or how has my health changed, if this is my first?

....
....
....
....
....

The specific tests I need:

....
....
....

Why?

....
....
....
....
....

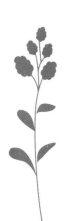

O Strawberry jam

O Peanut butter cups

O Mangos

O Pickles

O ....

O ....

O ....

O ....

O ....

O ....

My new cravings

The things I miss most

O Mojitos

O Sushi

O Hot dogs

O Fancy Brie

O ....

O ....

O ....

O ....

O ....

O ....

My Diet

What I had to give up

- ○ Coffee
- ○ Soda
- ○ Alcohol
- ○ Rare meats
- ○ Deli meats
- ○ Raw eggs
- ○ Raw fish
- ○ Smoked salmon
- ○ Raw shellfish
- ○ Unpasteurized cheeses
- ○ ....
- ○ ....
- ○ ....
- ○ ....
- ○ ....

Foods I can't stand right now

- ○ Milk
- ○ Garlic
- ○ Onions
- ○ Peppers
- ○ ....
- ○ ....
- ○ ....
- ○ ....
- ○ ....

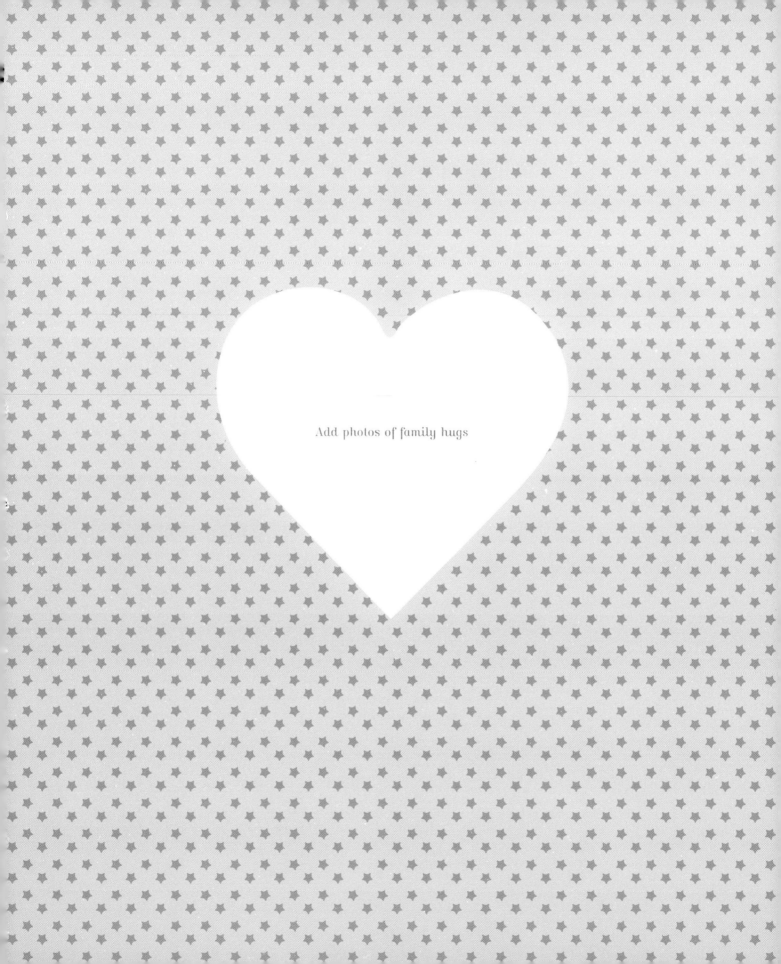

Add photos of family hugs

Our Connection

How I think this pregnancy may
change our relationship:

....
....
....
....
....

How I feel about this:

....
....
....
....
....

How he thinks this pregnancy may
change our relationship:

....
....
....
....
....

How he feels about this:

....
....
....
....
....

How we keep the spark alive:

....
....
....

My children's reactions to my big belly:

....
....
....

The changes that impress me most:

○ My ample cleavage   ○ My huge appetite

○ My skin's ability to stretch   ○ My bulging belly button

○ ....

○ ....

○ ....

○ ....

What I miss about my old body:

○ My stomach   ○ My energy level

○ My flawless skin   ○ My center of gravity

○ ....

○ ....

○ ....

○ ....

I'm taking care of my body by:

○ Keeping it moisturized   ○ Cutting out sweets

○ Exercising   ○ Giving myself pedicures

○ ....

○ ....

○ ....

○ ....

My Body

The new me, month after month

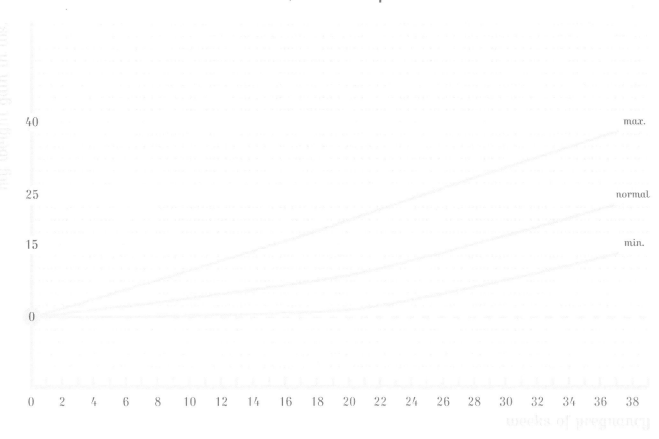

	my bra size	my pant size
Month 1		
Month 2		
Month 3		
Month 4		
Month 5		

	my bra size	my pant size
Month 6		
Month 7		
Month 8		
Month 9		

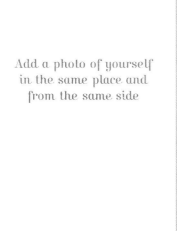

Add a photo of yourself
in the same place and
from the same side

Ninth month

My Growing Waist

Before getting pregnant:
.... in.

1st month: .... in.

2nd month: .... in.

3rd month: .... in.

4th month: .... in.

5th month: .... in.

6th month: .... in.

7th month: .... in.

8th month: .... in.

9th month: .... in.

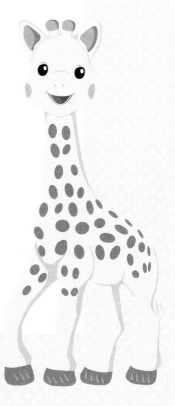

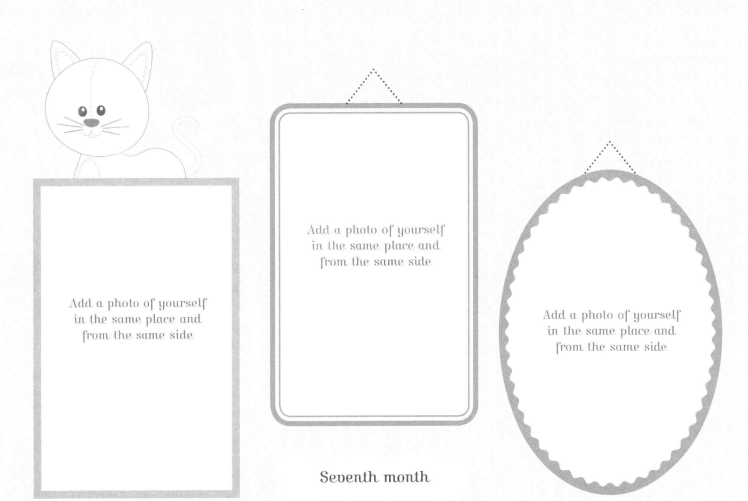

Add a photo of yourself
in the same place and
from the same side

Add a photo of yourself
in the same place and
from the same side

Add a photo of yourself
in the same place and
from the same side

Seventh month

Sixth month

Eighth month

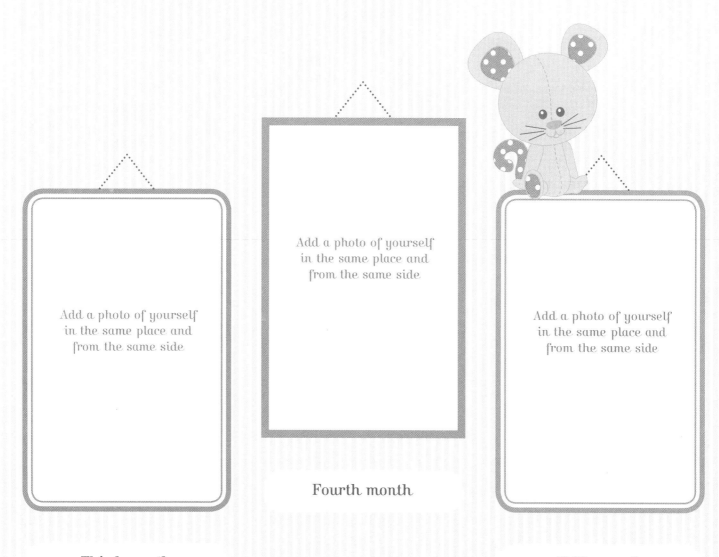

Add a photo of yourself
in the same place and
from the same side

Add a photo of yourself
in the same place and
from the same side

Add a photo of yourself
in the same place and
from the same side

Fourth month

Third month

Fifth month

My Growing Belly,
Month by Month

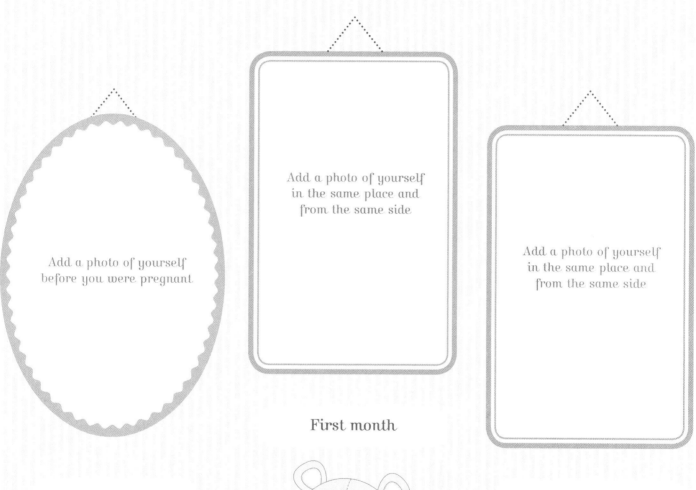

Add a photo of yourself
before you were pregnant

Add a photo of yourself
in the same place and
from the same side

Add a photo of yourself
in the same place and
from the same side

First month

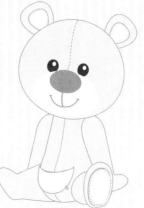

Pre-pregnancy

Second month

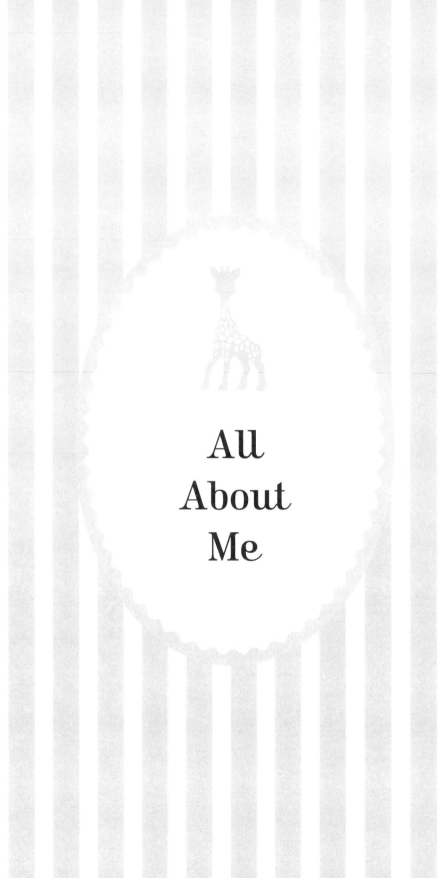

All
About
Me

Little things that bring me joy:

O A day at the spa with the girls
O My older children giving my belly a big hug
O Compliments on how I'm glowing
O Having someone offer me their seat
O My mother taking up knitting again
O My niece offering to babysit
O ....
O ....
O ....
O ....
O ....

Baby Gifts I've Received So Far

What?	From whom?	Comments
Sophie la girafe		

My Pregnancy in Public

Silly remarks people have made:

O You need to eat for two now

O You'll never lose all the baby weight

O No more watching horror movies

O Keep exercising—you're not sick

O Stop exercising—you'll hurt the baby

O ....

O ....

O ....

O ....

O ....

I hate it when people:

O Rub my belly without asking

O Treat me like an alien

O Ask nosy personal questions

O Watch me struggle with my huge bags on the subway

O Ask me if I'm due soon . . . at 4 months

O ....

O ....

O ....

O ....

O ....

What My Friends Said . . .

☺ Nice comments

Who? ....

What? ....

....

Who? ....

What? ....

....

Who? ....

What? ....

....

Who? ....

What? ....

....

Not-so-nice comments ☹

Who? ....

What? ....

....

Who? ....

What? ....

....

Who? ....

What? ....

....

Who? ....

What? ....

....

Telling My
Friends

Add a photo of you and your friends

Who did I tell first?

....

Why?

....

Their reaction?

....
....
....

Telling my in-laws

When? ....

Where? ....

How? ....
....

Their reaction:
....
....
....

What I thought of their reaction:
....
....
....
....

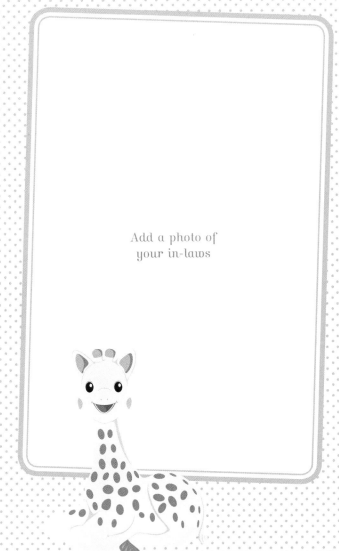

Add a photo of
your in-laws

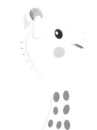

Telling the Future Grandparents

Telling my parents

When? ....

Where? ....

How? ....
....

Their reaction:
....
....
....

What I thought of their reaction:
....
....
....
....
....

Add a photo of
your parents

Spreading the Good News

The first time . . .

I dreamed about my baby

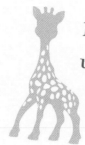

I noticed pregnant
women everywhere

The last time . . .

I drank alcohol

I could button my jeans

Add a photo of your first ultrasound

A memory I'll keep from this day:

....

....

....

....

My First Doctor's Visit

When is it?

....

Where is it?

....

Who's coming with me?

....

What are my concerns?

....

....

....

....

....

What I learned:

....

....

....

....

My reaction:

....

....

....

....

The reaction of the person who came with me:

....

....

....

....

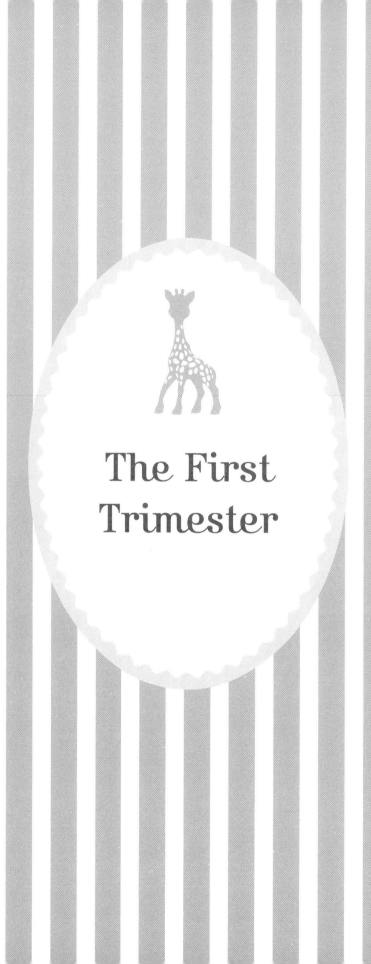

The First
Trimester

My favorite girl names:

....
....
....
....
....
....
....
....

My top choice:

....

My favorite boy names:

....
....
....
....
....
....
....
....

My top choice:

....

Our
Baby Name
Wishlists

His favorite girl names:

....
....
....
....
....
....
....
....

His top choice:

....

His favorite boy names:

....
....
....
....
....
....
....
....

His top choice:

....

Our shortlist for a girl:

....
....
....

Our shortlist for a boy:

....
....
....

Our Baby's Name

The names we chose

If it's a girl:

....

Who suggested this?................................

Why this name?...

....

....

....

....

What will her last name be?

....

....

Any middle names?

....

....

....

If it's a boy:

....

Who suggested this?................................

Why this name?...

....

....

....

....

What will his last name be?

....

....

Any middle names?

....

....

Traits we hope to pass on:

O My mom's delicate nose

O My dad's bright blue eyes

O My mother-in-law's smooth complexion

O My father-in-law's strong cheekbones

O ....

O ....

O ....

O ....

Traits we'd rather not pass on:

O My mom's near-sightedness

O My dad's large chin

O My mother-in-law's short stature

O My father-in-law's baldness

O ....

O ....

O ....

O ....

Us, when we were young

The starting points

Add a picture of
yourself as a baby

Add a picture of
Dad as a baby

Me

Dad

With the way our family looks,
our baby will probably have:

Hair:

○ Blond   ○ Red

○ Brown   ○ Straight

○ Black   ○ Curly

○ ....

Eyes:

○ Blue   ○ Hazel

○ Brown   ○ Gray

○ Green

○ ....

Personally, I think I'm having a:

Add a photo from
your last party

Our Last Holiday Alone

Our Last Big Party

Add a photo from your
last holiday alone together

....
....
....
....
....
....

....
....

Our Times Together

Add a photo of a time when
it was just the two of you

Add a photo of your
last time away together

Add a photo of your
last vacation alone together

WEEK

19 20

WEEK

23

His plan for the birth:

O He wants to be there for the entire experience

O He wants to be there at the beginning, but isn't
   sure he'll make it through

O He wants to cut the cord

O He wants to record everything

He also wants to ....
....
....
....

WEEK

27

WEEK

34

How I feel about all of this:

The nice surprises:

....
....
....
....
....
....
....
....
....
....
....
....
....
....

WEEK

38

The not-so-nice surprises:

....
....
....
....
....
....
....
....
....
....
....
....
....

From Week to Week

WEEK

1

WEEK

2

WEEK

3

His reaction to my changing body:

....
....
....
....

He's getting involved by:

○ Helping me watch my diet

○ Being extra affectionate

○ Coming to each ultrasound appointment

○ Joining me in birthing class

○ Turning the home office into the baby's room

He's also ....
....
....
....
....
....
....

WEEK

9

WEEK

10

His thoughtful gestures:

○ Giving me massages

○ Running all the errands

○ Making me his famous lasagna

○ Telling me I'm beautiful

○ Talking to my belly

Other considerate acts ....
....
....
....

WEEK

15

WEEK

17

WEEK

18

His worries:

....
....
....
....
....
....

His resolutions:

O Stop smoking

O Find a house with a big yard

O Get a promotion

O Start working out again

O ....

O ....

O ....

O ....

O ....

O ....

How I shared the news with my kids:

....
....
....
....
....

Their reaction:

....
....
....
....
....

The Announcement

How I told him the good news:

....
....
....
....
....
....

How he reacted:

....
....
....
....
....
....

What I thought of his reaction:

....
....
....
....
....
....

His hopes:

....
....
....
....
....

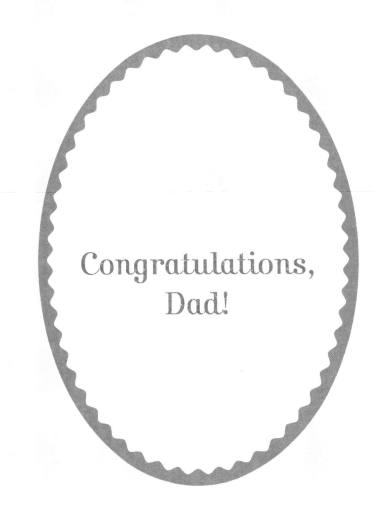

Congratulations,
Dad!

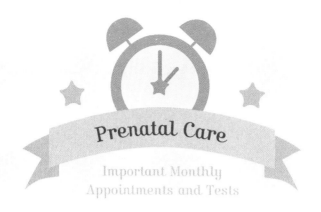

Prenatal Care

Important Monthly
Appointments and Tests

Months 1 and 2:

o See my doctor
o Get any tests I need
o Look into my employer's maternity leave policies
o Register with a birthing center
o Start thinking about a daycare service

Month 3:

o First prenatal visit
o Get any tests I need
o Find out if I'm eligible for short-term disability from my employer or my state
o Advise my employer
o Decide whether Dad will be taking time off, too
o First ultrasound (around 10 weeks of pregnancy, or 12 weeks after last menstrual period)

Month 4:

o Second prenatal visit
o Get any tests I need
o Determine if I've accrued any vacation, personal leave, or sick days to extend my leave

Month 5:

o Third prenatal visit
o Second ultrasound (around 22 weeks of pregnancy, or 24 weeks after last menstrual period)
o Find out about birthing classes and sign up as soon as possible

Month 6:

o Fourth prenatal visit
o Get any tests I need
o Sign up for daycare or find a nanny

Month 7:

o Fifth prenatal visit
o Get any tests I need
o If I'm considering unpaid leave, figure out how much time I can take
o Third ultrasound (around 30 weeks of pregnancy, or 32 weeks after last menstrual period)

Month 8:

o Sixth prenatal visit
o Get any tests I need
o Remember to officially request leave at least 30 days in advance
o Make a post-pregnancy work schedule
o Prepare my hospital bag and suitcase
o Organize babysitting for my older chidren for the big day

Month 9:

o Seventh prenatal visit
o Get any tests I need
o Meet with the anesthesiologist